"*The Hero's Mask* tells the story of children becoming heroes! It will inspire all who read it to face and overcome challenges with courage and bravery. *The Hero's Mask* is not about what has happened to you but who you can become. *The Hero's Mask Guidebook* combines research on the impact of trauma with a magical unfolding of the individual uniqueness and beauty of each child. It integrates theory, knowledge, and evidence-based practice with a soul depth that transcends the moment and calls us to be our 'best' selves to children. It provides a sacred pathway for child, parent, and adult healing."
James Henry, Ph.D. Professor of Social Work and Project Director, Children's Trauma Assessment Center, Western Michigan University.

"In the tradition of Joseph Campbell, George Lucas, and J.K. Rowling, Dr. Kagan uses the stories of heroes to illustrate how children can go through difficult times, learn from past mistakes, find strength in friendship, cope with the fear, discomfort, and paralysis of traumatic reminders, and become heroes in their own lives. He also illustrates in very practical ways how adults can nurture a child's inner resilience by showing grace and compassion, guiding them to shape their own narrative and make heroic choices. In *The Hero's Mask*, Dr. Kagan tells a story that children will love, full of mystery and friendship, bullies and heroism. Through that story children can relate to a hero in Carrie, whose relationships help her to overcome her fears and understand the strength she and her friends have to make a difference in other's lives. Through Carrie's story, children can understand the power of connection and engagement as paths towards healing and heroism."
Jane Halladay Goldman, Ph.D., Director, Service Systems Program, UCLA-Duke University National Center for Child Traumatic Stress.

"*The Hero's Mask* is an engaging and timely novel about the impact of traumatic loss on children and much of what it takes for them to heal: good friends, nurturing adults, cultural wisdom, personal courage—and the power of storytelling itself. The companion *Guidebook* is a rich resource for caregivers, teachers, and counselors wanting to engage in deeper understanding and the difficult conversations that can support children through these toughest times."

Martha B. Straus, Ph.D., Professor, Antioch University and author of *Treating Trauma in Adolescents: Development, Attachment, and the Therapeutic Relationship.*

"In his novel, *The Hero's Mask*, Dr. Kagan beautifully demonstrates the profound power of connection in promoting healing and resilience. Through his characters and the theme of a hero's journey, he is able to bring the thematic of loss, human stress and the role of relationship to life in a context that is relatable to young people and the caregivers who support them. This novel along with the practical guidebook for parents and professionals is a unique tool written by someone who has clearly dedicated a career to understanding trauma, attachment, resilience and young people! Youth serving systems, families and children alike will benefit from this approach."

Kristine M. Kinniburgh, LCSW, Director of Trauma Services, Justice Resource Institute Connecticut, National trauma trainer and consultant, The Trauma Center at JRI. ARC Co-Developer and Co-author of *Treating traumatic stress in children and adolescents; How to foster resilience through attachment, self-regulation, and competency* (Guilford Press).

"*The Hero's Mask* is a very engaging, age-appropriate, and inspiring novel for middle grade children, especially for those who have experienced traumatic losses, bullying, disengaged parents and harsh authority figures. The central characters are multi-dimensional and relatable, and the narrative moves forward in an adept, fast-paced manner that will engage most young readers. *The Hero's Mask* and the accompanying *Guidebook* represent a significant contribution to an understanding of children's trauma and actions that can be taken to reduce and resolve trauma."

Cheryl Lanktree, Ph.D., Adolescent Trauma Training Center, Keck School of Medicine, University of Southern California.

"For children and young teens who are feeling a lot of big emotions and are struggling to be understood, follow Carrie, the "hero" of *The Hero's Mask*, as she puts the feelings shared by so many others into words. This novel beautifully describes the way stress and trauma can show up in our bodies and affect our relationships with family and peers. Young readers learn with Carrie as she begins to connect the dots between her thoughts, feelings, and behaviors—to change the direction of her own story for the better. *The Hero's Mask* is a great resource for schools that illustrates what students are really experiencing, how this affects their ability to learn and their behavior in the classroom, and the transformative role that educators can play. The accompanying Guidebook provides educators with a framework for understanding trauma-informed schools, as well as a structured approach for using *The Hero's Mask* with students in the classroom."

Jenifer Maze, PhD, Deputy Director, UCLA-Duke University National Center for Child Traumatic Stress.

"In writing *The Hero's Mask* and *Helping Children with Traumatic Stress*, Dr. Kagan offers a gift to children and families who have experienced trauma and to the caregivers, educators, and therapists who support these families. *The Hero's Mask* works as a standalone piece of literature with its well-developed characters and salient themes of interpersonal, community, and cultural adversity, trauma, and loss. Through 11-year-old Carrie and the other children and adults in her life, many readers will identify with the somatic, emotional, and behavioral experiences associated with trauma and will gain a narrative of hope, possibility, and healing through connection. *Helping Children with Traumatic Stress*, a companion resource to *The Hero's Mask*, offers accessible evidence-informed tools to support children and families in their journey of healing from trauma. Caregivers, educators, and therapists will find the curriculum guide with its specific objectives and activities invaluable in supporting connections with children and in providing developmentally-appropriate, culturally-sensitive, trauma-informed care."

Mindy Kronenberg, Ph.D., IMH-E®, Clinical Psychologist and Adjunct Professor, University of Memphis, Co-Editor of *Treating Traumatized Children: A Casebook of Evidence-based Therapies*.

"Brilliant psychoeducation on trauma, resilience and the power of relationships disguised as a middle grade novel. Reading *The Hero's Mask* together should stimulate supportive and healing discussions between middle schoolers and their adult mentors. Overall a wonderful therapeutic resource!"

Laurel J. Kiser, Ph.D., M.B.A., Associate Professor, Division of Psychiatric Services Research, Department of Psychiatry, University of Maryland School of Medicine.

"*The Hero's Mask*, written by a national expert in child traumatic stress, creatively addresses important ways educators, professionals, and caregivers can support a child dealing with pain from trauma and adversity. The *Guidebook* follows along with the novel as Carrie, our middle school role model, engages us with her courage and personality in facing overwhelming feelings, trauma triggers, and broken connections with family and peers that often occur when trauma and grief impact our youth. Kagan's text offer guidance and inspiration to important adults in children's lives to use the power of their relationships in informed, healing, and transformative ways."

Lisa Amaya-Jackson, MD, MPH, Deputy Director, UCLA-Duke National Center for Child Traumatic Stress.

"*The Hero's Mask* books go beyond the growing awareness of ACES and provide practical tools that concerned parents, teachers, counselors and therapists can use to rebuild the emotionally supportive relationships children need to thrive after experiences of hardship and trauma. The novel engages children and caring adults to experience adversity through the eyes of a child including what can help and what can hurt a troubled child. The *Guidebook* provides a curriculum for exploration of heroes that can help children, classrooms and schools to take steps to prevent or reduce traumatic stress. Together, these books provide essential resources for trauma-informed schools and programs."

Heather Larkin Halloway, Ph.D., Associate Professor, School of Social Welfare, State University of New York at Albany.

"Richard Kagan weaves together story with trauma-informed principles and interventions. As the reader learns about Carrie, her history, her challenges, and her strengths, they are learning important lessons about stress and trauma that they can apply to themselves or those around them. His metaphor of the mask is powerful, and through story, he offers dialogues about heroes, fear and how it affects us, the importance of taking a stand, reaching out for support, and showing up as your authentic self. These dialogues are core to both trauma treatments and trauma-informed systems, and it is refreshing to see them embraced in a story. Children, parents, and teachers will benefit from reading The Hero's Mask, and I strongly believe it will help them open doors to important conversations that lead to healing."

Chandra Ghosh Ippen, Ph.D., Associate Director, Child Trauma Research Program, University of California, San Francisco.

The Hero's Mask Guidebook: Helping Children with Traumatic Stress

The Hero's Mask Guidebook provides practical strategies to be used alongside the *The Hero's Mask* novel. *The Guidebook* has been designed to promote an understanding of the impact of traumatic stress and what counselors, therapists, educators, parents and caregivers can do to promote healing and recovery. *The Guidebook* and storybook can be used together to spark conversations around the difficult topics of loss and trauma and to create openings for renewing and strengthening emotionally supportive relationships with distressed children after traumatic experiences.

The *Guidebook* identifies resources to access information about treatment programs and strategies that can help children and families with traumatic stress and integration of *The Hero's Mask* books with *Real Life Heroes*®, an evidence-supported treatment program for children and families with traumatic stress.

Richard Kagan is a clinical psychologist and the author and co-author of 12 books and 35+ articles, chapters, and papers on practice and research issues in trauma therapy, child welfare, foster care, adoption, professional development, program evaluation, and quality improvement in family service and behavioral health care programs. Dr. Kagan's publications highlight practical and innovative approaches that counselors, therapists, educators, parents and caregivers can utilize to help children and families strengthen resilience and reduce traumatic stress.

The Hero's Mask Guidebook: Helping Children with Traumatic Stress

A Resource for Educators, Counselors, Therapists, Parents and Caregivers

Richard Kagan

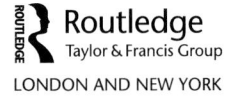

Routledge
Taylor & Francis Group

LONDON AND NEW YORK

First published 2021
by Routledge
2 Park Square, Milton Park, Abingdon, Oxon OX14 4RN

and by Routledge
52 Vanderbilt Avenue, New York, NY 10017

Routledge is an imprint of the Taylor & Francis Group, an informa business

© 2021 Richard Kagan

The right of Richard Kagan to be identified as author of this work has been asserted by him in accordance with sections 77 and 78 of the Copyright, Designs and Patents Act 1988.

All rights reserved. No part of this book may be reprinted or reproduced or utilised in any form or by any electronic, mechanical, or other means, now known or hereafter invented, including photocopying and recording, or in any information storage or retrieval system, without permission in writing from the publishers.

Trademark notice: Product or corporate names may be trademarks or registered trademarks, and are used only for identification and explanation without intent to infringe.

British Library Cataloguing-in-Publication Data
A catalogue record for this book is available from the British Library

Library of Congress Cataloging-in-Publication Data
Names: Kagan, Richard, author.
Title: The hero's mask guidebook : helping children with traumatic stress : a resource for educators, counselors, therapists, parents and caregivers / Richard Kagan.
Description: Abingdon, Oxon ; New York, NY : Routledge, 2021. | Includes bibliographical references.
Identifiers: LCCN 2020019134 (print) | LCCN 2020019135 (ebook) | ISBN 9780367474294 (paperback) | ISBN 9781003035541 (ebook)
Subjects: LCSH: Psychic trauma in children--Treatment--Handbooks, manuals, etc.
Classification: LCC RJ506.P66 P334 2021 (print) | LCC RJ506.P66 (ebook) | DDC 618.92/852106--dc23
LC record available at https://lccn.loc.gov/2020019134
LC ebook record available at https://lccn.loc.gov/2020019135

ISBN: 978-0-367-47429-4 (pbk)
ISBN: 978-1-003-03554-1 (ebk)

Typeset in AntitledBook
by MPS Limited, Dehradun

In memory of Rhoda and Fred Kagan

Contents

Preface

In my work as a clinical psychologist, children have shared with me traumatic experiences that ripped their families apart and shattered their sense of trust and belonging. These same children have also shared with me a yearning to be loved and the courage to change. I have been inspired by how children recovered from losses of the family members they loved, emotional, physical and sexual abuse, family violence, neglect, and abandonments. I have also seen how many children remained mired in the nightmares of their lives and appeared to relive their greatest fears day after day. Many children appeared cut off from emotionally supportive relationships with caring adults and appeared to repeat the abuse and violence they had experienced in their own behaviors. Dangerous behaviors led to referrals to child welfare services, juvenile justice programs, psychiatric hospitals or behavioral health care programs.

My job as a psychologist was to engage these children and their families and to find a way to understand what had happened and what could be done to help them. Rather than viewing these children as helpless victims or frightening aggressors, I learned to listen and watch for clues to what made these children smile as well as what led to dangerous behaviors. From these children, their parents, caregivers, and my colleagues, I learned lessons about what could be done to transform their lives. I also learned how their stories of trauma and recovery could inspire all of us.

Each child and family I have worked with has taught me a lesson of how ordinary people can rise up to surmount tragedies. Very often, the worst traumas involved the breakdown of a child's trust in parents, guardians, and other adults to keep themselves and their families safe. Many children appeared cut off from emotionally supportive relationships with caring adults and appeared to repeat the abuse and violence they had experienced in their own behaviors. Parents, grandparents, teachers, counselors and other caring adults often felt threatened by what children did and said after multiple traumas. Caring adults often felt disempowered and unable to re-connect with troubled children. At the same time, troubled children often felt increasingly alone and desperate with little hope.

I wrote *The Hero's Mask* to create openings for parents, teachers, therapists, and other caring adults to encourage children to share what may be hidden from adults—what makes them smile, what they yearn for, who they admire, and what drives their fears. Children read stories and connect with feelings of characters like themselves facing real-life problems like the death of a parent, parents' fighting, financial problems, or school bullies. And these stories of facing and overcoming problems can, in turn, renew hope and bring out children's drive to learn skills and make things better. In the same way, books can remind adults how they can become the heroes children need to face unspoken terrors and to learn to grow and thrive again after experiencing adversity. In this way, books like The Hero's Mask can help children and caring adults repair frayed bonds and recover from losses and other stressful experiences.

This *Guidebook* includes suggestions and guidelines for how parents, caregivers, educators, counselors and therapists can use *The Hero's Mask* novel to help the children they love. The Guidebook also includes resources and references to find additional information about helping children and families with traumatic stress and use of Real Life Heroes® (RLH), an evidence-supported treatment program for children and families with traumatic stress. *The Real Life Heroes Toolkit for Treating Traumatic Stress in Children and Families*, 2nd Edn (Routledge, 2017), *The Real Life Heroes Life Storybook*, 3rd Edn (Routledge, 2017) and *Rebuilding Attachments with Traumatized Children* (Routledge, 2004) provide an integrated framework for use of RLH in trauma- and resiliency-focused treatment and development of trauma-informed schools and treatment programs.[1] For additional stories of children with traumatic stress and the lessons they can teach us, please see *Wounded Angels, Inspiration from Children in Crisis*, 2nd Edn (Routledge, 2017). *The Hero's Mask* and RLH books can be used to promote an understanding of trauma and to strengthen (or develop) attunement and emotionally supportive relationships between children and caring adults and resilience to traumatic stress in families, schools and communities.

Richard Kagan

Note

1 For additional information about *Real Life Heroes*®, please see www.reallifeheroes.net.

1. Promoting awareness of traumatic stress and what can be done to help children, families and schools

ACES

Adverse childhood experiences (ACES)[1] and toxic or traumatic stress[2] have been recognized as critical public health problems linked with impaired development of children's abilities to focus attention, to learn at school, to manage stress, and to the development of mental and physical health disorders, addictions, and high-risk behavior problems. Traumatic stress impacts all communities from large cities to villages, suburbs, and rural areas. Traumatic experiences can damage the security, caring and guidance children need to grow and thrive. Children show symptoms of traumatic stress when they lose trust in adults in their families, schools, and communities to maintain safety, nurture, and guidance.

Parents, caregivers, educators, and other caring adults have the power to prevent many adverse childhood experiences and to help children recover from traumas, but to do that often means addressing difficult issues that many people try to avoid. Improving the lives of children, caregivers, and communities begins with becoming aware of how childhood experiences of deaths, severe illness, parents fighting, parental unavailability, emotional, physical or sexual abuse, abandonment, racism, natural disasters, bullies, violence in the child's home or neighborhood, and other highly stressful events can alter children's capacity to regulate their emotions, focus attention, manage behaviors, learn vital skills, and succeed at school and later as adults.

Traumatic stress

Children (and adults) can develop symptoms of toxic or traumatic stress when they experience events that they perceive as threatening severe harm or death to themselves or someone they love and when a child or adult lacks the ability and supportive relationships to manage these threats. Adverse childhood experiences can lead to traumatic stress reactions dysregulation and behavior problems.

When a child feels their lives and the lives of those they love are no longer safe, the child may develop long-lasting changes in how they think, feel, or respond with their bodies. Children's heart rates may increase and they may begin to sweat, become agitated, feel tense, feel aches or pains or 'butterflies in their stomachs,' and become hyper alert. After a traumatic event, children may watch and listen vigilantly for signs that scary or dangerous things could happen again. Children may become emotionally upset with little warning in reaction to sounds, smells, or other reminders of past traumas that are not noticed by other children or adults. They may react by withdrawing, isolating, running away, getting into fights, or angrily lashing out at other children or adults.

Traumatic stress reactions are often very distressing, but, in fact, these reactions are also very normal. Our bodies protect us and prepare us to survive dangers. At the same time, these reactions can interfere with children' physical and emotional health, especially if they have experienced multiple traumas that were unpredictable or disrupted children's relationships and security with caregivers. Children cannot learn or develop important social skills when they are always on the lookout for danger and when their bodies are ready to react quickly to any perception of risk for the child, family members, or other people the child loves. Attention and memory problems are common reactions along with difficulty making plans or solving problems. Children with traumatic stress may fall behind in school and lack the ability to manage common requests by caregivers, teachers, or others in the community leading to increased conflicts. Symptoms often include intense and ongoing emotional upset and agitation, chronic anxiety, behavioral changes, difficulties maintaining attention, school problems, nightmares, physical symptoms such as difficulty sleeping and eating, or symptoms of depression.

Traumatic stress may appear in different ways with different children. Reactions are often related to the child's age, ability to understand, ability to cope, and feelings of security in their relationships with caregivers at the time that traumatic events occurred. One child in a family may react much more strongly than another child, often depending on their ability to cope, emotional maturity, and the support they experience during and after traumatic events.

The good news is that parents and caregivers can help the children they care about by rebuilding emotionally attuned relationships and modeling how to build strengths and the courage to face hard times and make things better. Parents and caring adults can also access evidence-supported treatments have been developed that can help children and their families who are suffering from traumatic stress.

The Hero's Mask

The Hero's Mask captures the experience of Carrie, a fifth-grade girl, grappling with the loss of her father and grandmother, job losses and economic decline in her city, her mother's depression, bullies, and a harsh teacher aide. The book traces Carrie's discovery of strengths within herself and her family and how she benefits from developing relationships with friends and caring adults. Together, with help from her friends, mother, teachers, and a neighbor, Carrie's story demonstrates how families can get through hard times similar to the experiences that many American children face today.

The Hero's Mask engages readers to recognize how traumatic stress works, to confront sensitive issues, and, most important, to understand what can be done to make things better. In the course of the story, Carrie experiences symptoms of traumatic stress and learns more effective ways to cope. The book highlights Carrie's growing awareness of her own emotional reactions to stressful events in her family, school and community, the reactions of family members, peers, teachers, and school leaders, and what helps to make their lives better.

Carrie, her family and friends struggle with experiences that have challenged many families, especially after economic recessions, a pandemic and increasing difficulties for many parents/caregivers to manage work needed to financially support their families and, at the same time, to provide the time and care needed to raise children. *The Hero's Mask* can be used in families, schools and health care programs to open up conversations about healing from traumatic stress. Reading *The Hero's Mask* can help bring children and adults together to support each other in 'tough times' and overcome challenges and obstacles that have threatened families, schools, and communities. Parents and other caring adults can use the story to help their children understand factors leading to traumatic stress, how this can lead to behavioral problems at home and in school, and what can be done to help.

This is a book about bridging gaps between children, parents and other caregivers that can develop during 'tough times.' Through Carrie, the book portrays a girl's transition to greater awareness of what drives behaviors by her parents and educators, how mentors can promote children's development, and the power of reclaiming a distressed child. Parents, grandparents, a teacher, and a principal take on important roles in helping Carrie develop an understanding of how fears inhibit children and adults, and how friendships and supportive adults can foster the courage to take risks and make things better. *The Hero's Mask* is a story of overcoming, of real-life heroes in a small city, and, most of all, about the power of caring to promote resilience.

Developmental level

The Hero's Mask is intended for children with a fourth–sixth grade reading level, their parents and other caring adults concerned with traumatic stress. Latency is a critical age to help traumatized children and their families overcome obstacles to development and increase feelings of belonging, trust in caregivers, and skills for managing stress before adolescence when high-risk behaviors may increase. The book is also useful for adolescents who function cognitively, emotionally or socially at a younger developmental level. Many adolescents who have experienced multiple traumas and disrupted attachments appear delayed in their social, emotional, and cognitive development and function at a level more typical of latency-age children.

Empowering parents and caregivers

Parents and caregivers can use *The Hero's Mask* to show children that they are able to talk about difficult or painful experiences that may be hard to bring up in families, and that together, caring adults and children can make things better. Reading, or talking about the book together, provides an opportunity for children, parents, and other caring adults to re-connect or to build new and emotionally supportive relationships. The book can help *adults* talk with children about 'tough times' the adults have experienced in a way that is not overwhelming to children and which does not involve details that children are unable to manage. Adults can share how they had felt vulnerable in 'tough times' and highlight the lessons they and other family members learned that helped them survive and grow stronger. In this way, caring adults can demonstrate that it is okay to talk about 'tough times' and to model how adults and children can get through traumatic experiences and build better lives.

This is a book about how families can come together, heal strained relationships, and overcome challenges. The book highlights the central role of parents, teachers, and other caring adults to help children thrive and how families and communities can grow stronger from generation to generation. In this way, parents and caregivers can help children to incorporate strengths in their families and cultural heritage for managing adversity.

Challenges addressed in *The Hero's Mask*

The Hero's Mask builds on the work of Joseph Campbell[3] to highlight growth and mastery by everyday people experiencing hardships and imagery from the 'heroes journey' that can inspire facing and reducing the power of traumatic memories. Over the course of the book, Carrie learns how masks can help and also make things worse, how masks can be used to hide feelings and avoid facing hardships or painful memories, how to recognize when other people are using masks, and the importance of owning your own mask and controlling when to use your mask. For Carrie, this is framed by her need to figure out what happened in her family and community and her frustration with adults who appear unable to face or share the truth about what happened.

The Hero's Mask portrays how children will strive to take control when they experience adults avoiding facing hardships and traumatic experiences. This can lead to what adults see as disrespect, sneaking around adults or defiance, followed by harsher discipline by adults who seek to restore control without addressing underlying problems. Harsher discipline, in turn, can lead to greater separation of children from the parents, caregivers, teachers, and other caring adults they need.

The Hero's Mask provides an antidote for this negative cycle by encouraging caring adults to learn from children and by illustrating how children's behaviors can be used by caring adults to uncover central challenges that need to be resolved. In many ways, traumatized children can be seen as wounded angels lighting a pathway for caring adults to unspoken terrors that continue to afflict children, families and communities.[4] Caring adults can follow these pathways to help their children, their families and communities to heal and to restore the role of caring adults as protectors, guides and leaders.

Tough times and adverse experiences addressed in the book include: managing the strain of declining incomes and lost jobs, grieving the loss of a father and a grandmother, coping with a parent or relative's feelings of depression after multiple losses, helping students and schools confront bullying by peers, protecting students from harsh discipline, and helping students and teachers manage increasing pressures to achieve on standardized testing. Parents, caregivers, and teachers can use the book to discuss with their children:

- The impact of deaths, job losses, bullying, and other forms of adversity and what makes a stressful experiences become traumatic.
- What children and caring adults can do to help each other and prevent traumatic stress including signaling each other if they sense danger.
- What can help children and adults who have experienced trauma grow stronger than tough times.
- How families, schools and communities can protect children from bullying and harsh discipline and promote learning vital skills for resilience during tough times.

Promoting healing with storytelling

Stories stimulate children and adults to experience what characters are going through and to share in characters' discovery of what is hard and what can help. Stories evoke curiosity, and, curiosity stimulates new learning, growth, and finding ways to get beyond the nightmares of the past.

Stories can also provide a means of opening up conversations about subjects that have been suppressed. Children (and caregivers) often become engrossed in stories of children (and adults) who face similar problems as themselves, even when they are not willing to talk about their own traumatic experiences, read guides to learning about traumas or utilize self-help workbooks designed to develop coping skills. Stories create a distance that allows children (and caregivers) to think about traumas in a way that is not so threatening that they generate painful or overwhelming feelings of distress. Reading fiction also helps youths separate themselves from reminders of shame about what they have done, or not done, that may be linked to traumatic memories. In psychotherapy, fictionalized stories, like *The Hero's Mask*, open the door to addressing critical treatment issues in a way that is manageable and sustains engagement in trauma treatment.

The Hero's Mask appeals to middle grade readers as a mystery that children in the story uncover including secrets about a teacher's sudden departure, a missing baby rat and a principal's role in what is happening in a school. At a deeper level, the book invites children and caregivers to learn what drives Carrie's behaviors, including the impact of losing her father and feeling like her mother no longer cares. Reading about Carrie and her friends evokes children's natural drive to figure out what is going on and to make things better for the people they care about.

Highlighting strengths

Focusing on building or increasing strengths modeled after heroes encourages learning new skills to overcome problems and learning from the experiences of family members who have learned how to survive adversity. Thinking about heroes also evokes hope for change.

Through Carrie, children (and parents/caregivers) can learn about the secrets behind masks that children and adults use to cope with hard times and what can increase the courage needed to take risks. *The Hero's Mask* demonstrates the importance of helping others and getting help for oneself as part of acting like a hero. Exploration of the secrets of heroes can be utilized with children and parents/caregivers in treatment programs to develop motivation for building coping skills, helping each other, mobilizing courage to find out 'what happened' that led up to traumatic stress, sharing 'what happened,' and developing safety plans to prevent repetition of traumas.

Cautionary note

Storytelling promotes healing through images and metaphors that evoke strengths and aspirations as well as stressful memories and fears. The power of storytelling comes from letting the metaphors and images in the story open up possibilities for healing,[5] for re-looking at the past in a safe way and re-envisioning opportunities for making a better future. It is important for parents, teachers and other caring adults to let the images and metaphors in the story move children to explore rather than forcing children to directly address traumatic events[6] or other difficulties when they may lack the trust and safety they need.

Children should not be required to read this book with adults they cannot trust to respect their feelings, keep them safe, validate children's traumatic experiences, protect children from becoming overwhelmed by the adult's own stress, or work to prevent recurrence of past traumas. Use of this book is also not recommended with children who are actively suicidal, violent, or psychotic or children at imminent risk of becoming self-abusive, suicidal, violent or engaging in life-threatening behaviors. Educators, counselors, therapists and other professionals should also be familiar with disclosure requirements if children (or parents/caregivers) share abuse, neglect, violence or risks of harm to themselves or others that must be reported.

Reading books like *The Hero's Mask* can open up opportunities for parents, teachers, and other caring adults to show children that they are able and willing to talk about tough times including traumatic experiences and to make necessary changes in their families, schools and communities to restore safety and security. This can help children to feel safe enough to share previously hidden experiences and work with parents, caregivers and therapists to grow stronger than their fears. At the same time, reading books is not a *substitute for working with a certified therapist to help children and families with traumatic stress*. Suggestions for when to involve a trauma therapist are provided in the next section.

Notes

1 Felitti, V.J., Anda, R.F., Nordenberg, D., Williamson, D.F., Spitz, A.M., Edwards, V., ... Marks, J.S. (1998). Relationship of childhood abuse and household dysfunction to many of the leading causes of death in adults. The adverse childhood experience study. *American Journal of Preventive Medicine*, *14*(4), 245–258.
2 Please see Shonkoff, J.P., Garner, A.S., and The Committee on Psychosocial Aspects of Child and Family Health, Committee on Early Childhood, Adoption, and Dependent Care, and Section on Developmental and Behavioral Pediatrics (2012). The lifelong effects of early childhood adversity and traumatic stress, *Pediatrics*, 2011–2663, 129, 232–246. doi:10.1542/peds.2011-2663 for a summary of research on toxic stress.
3 Campbell, J. (1968). *The Hero with a Thousand Faces*. Princeton, NJ: Princeton University Press.
4 Please see Kagan, R. (2017). *Wounded Angels; Inspiration from Children in Crisis*. New York: Routledge.
5 Anonymous Routledge reviewer.
6 Ibid.

2. Suggestions for use by parents and caregivers

Reading the book

The Hero's Mask can be read together with children or separately. Reading together provides natural segues for parents and caregivers to demonstrate that they can manage stressful experiences and are able and willing to help their children. If children prefer to read separately, it is important for parents and caregivers to show that they are also reading the book, thinking about issues addressed and want to help their children. Either way, parents and caregivers need to demonstrate to their children that they are committed to loving, protecting and guiding their children no matter what happened, how distressing this has been or what children have done.

Leading the way

Children naturally look to their parents, grandparents, aunts, uncles, and other caregivers to protect them and restore safety after 'tough times' including losses, injuries, violence, or natural disasters. Parents and caregivers can help their families overcome traumatic stress by developing an understanding of how trauma works and the supports and confidence they need to show children they can face what may appear to children to be overwhelming terrors. Parents and caregivers can model what courage means in their families and pass on stories of how family members have faced and overcame adversity. Sharing stories of overcoming can help children feel safe to share their own experiences when they felt afraid or were threatened or hurt. Parents and caregivers and can also encourage children to ask questions about things that happened that may be hard to talk about, e.g. the death of a family member. This can open up opportunities to help children to resolve problems and reduce stressors that have been interfering with their growth and development.

In sharing these stories, it is important that caring adults share experiences and lessons learned in ways that children can manage at their developmental level (understanding, reasoning, problem-solving, emotional regulation and social skills) and to avoid sharing experiences that can overwhelm children with fears for the safety of parents, other people or themselves. Children will watch adults to see if adults can remain modulated while sharing what happened and what was done to restore safety. Children need to know that parents and caregivers will be okay, especially if they have experienced the loss of another parent or caregivers or felt rejected or abandoned by parents or caregivers. It is very important that parents and other caregivers highlight what helped them get through 'tough times' and how they and others have taken steps to protect everyone from 'tough times' happening again.

It is also important that parents and other caregivers share their experiences while remaining sufficiently modulated so that children will not fear parents or caregivers becoming out of control or at risk of hurting themselves or other people, or rejecting or abandoning children. Parents and other caregivers need to demonstrate that they can remain emotionally available to children and committed to protecting, guiding and caring for their families. Consulting a therapist (see below) can help parents do this in a safe way that increases children's feelings of security and resilience when parents and caregivers feel that traumatic memories in their own lives or their children's lives could be overwhelming for them to share or that they cannot do this in a way that children can understand or manage.

Creating safety to share

Parents and caregivers create safety in their homes by establishing routines from getting up in the morning to stories and hugs at bedtime, and by maintaining these routines even after 'tough times.' Parents and caregivers also create safety by demonstrating that they will validate children's experiences including their feelings and can manage dealing with distressing experiences, feelings and what children have done in reaction to these experiences.

Parents can caregivers make it safe to share feelings by modeling how to do this through words, drawing, music, movement and rituals linked to their family's cultural heritage. Parents and caregivers can encourage children to share feelings nonverbally through art, rhythm, music, movement, and writing stories. In doing this, it is important that parents and caregivers let children feel in control of how they share feelings, rather than feeling forced to share thoughts or feelings in a proscribed way that leads them to feel inhibited, inadequate or even more out of control after experiencing a loss or 'tough time.'

Parents and caregivers can also encourage children to keep memories through journals, photo books, scrap books and memorials that are shared only with safe family members and other caring adults children can trust. Life story work is also valuable to help see traumatic events in the context of a full life and to help children to learn to grow stronger after experiencing adversity.

Utilizing resources for families who have experienced traumatic stress

For guides to talking with children about traumatic grief, please see:

www.nctsn.org/resources/the-power-of-parenting-how-to-help-your-child-after-a-parent-or-caregiver-dies, www.nctsn.org/trauma-types/traumatic-grief/parents-caregivers

www.nctsn.org/sites/default/files/assets/pdfs/helping_children_with_traumatic_grief.pdf

Support for families experiencing grief and loss can also be found at:

The Trauma and Grief Center: www.texaschildrens.org/departments/trauma-and-grief-center;
The National Alliance for Grieving Children: https://childrengrieve.org
NY Life Foundation: www.newyorklife.com/foundation/bereavement
The Family Bereavement Program: http://reachinstitute.asu.edu/programs/resilientparent

For younger children, *Samantha Jane's Missing Smile* (Magination Press) is a beautiful story about helping a child who experienced the loss of a parent including tips for parents and caregivers on helping children with grief.

Parents can learn more about traumatic stress, effective treatments for traumatic stress and parenting strategies from a number of sources including free downloadable guides from the National Child Traumatic Stress Network (NCTSN) at www.nctsn.org. For an introduction to understanding childhood traumatic stress, please see:

http://nctsn.org/sites/default/files/assets/pdfs/ctte_parents.pdf

For a resource guide to helping youths with Complex Trauma, please see:

www.nctsn.org/sites/default/files/assets/pdfs/ct_guide_final.pdf

For more information on adverse childhood experiences, please see:

www.npr.org/blogs/health/2015/03/02/377569413/can-family-secrets-make-yousick?utm_source=
facebook.com&utm_medium=social&utm_campaign=npr&utm_term=nprnews&utm_content=20150302

For additional resources on recognizing symptoms of traumatic stress, helping children following traumatic events, and finding evidence-supported treatments that can help children and families recover after traumas, please see:

www.nctsn.org/resources/audiences/parents-caregivers#q3

The NCTSN also provides a curriculum for grandparents, kinship, foster and adoptive parents, and legal guardians to make sense of their child's sometimes confusing feelings, attitudes, and behaviors and to use that understanding to help them cope with traumatic experiences. The NCTSN Resource Parent Curriculum, *Caring for Children Who Have Experienced Trauma: A Workshop for Resource Parents* is a free PowerPoint-based training curriculum. It provides foster, adoptive, and kinship parents with practical tools and information handouts to help their children move forward from their traumatic pasts, to recognize and reduce the impact of their children's traumas on themselves, and to seek useful support from others. To access the curriculum, please see:

www.nctsnet.org/products/caring-for-children-who-have-experienced-trauma

Information on trauma treatment models and research on traumatic grief is included in Chapter 6 of this *Guidebook*.

When should therapists be involved?

Professional therapists (licensed psychologists, psychiatrists, social workers, or mental health counselors) should be consulted when children show significant social, emotional, academic, or behavioral problems and don't improve with the support of parents, family members, mentors and friends or show severe symptoms or behaviors that create risks for themselves or others. Therapists should also be consulted when children do not feel safe to share their experiences with their parents or primary caregivers, when parents and primary caregivers feel they would become overwhelmed if they shared stories of overcoming or when parents and caregivers are not able to do this in a way that matches children's capacity to understand and remain feeling safe and secure in their primary relationships.

Therapists can play a critical role when children and parents or caregivers have conflicting memories of what happened. Children often experience events in different ways than adults because of their developmental level and the impact of previous experiences. Therapists can help parents and caregivers to bridge gaps that may have formed and reduce parent-child conflicts[1]. Therapists can also guide use of life story work through use of resources including the *Real Life Heroes Life Storybook*, 3rd Edn (Routledge) and the *Real Life Heroes Toolkit for Treating Traumatic Stress in Children and Families*, 2nd Edn by the author of *The Hero's Mask*.

Finding a trauma and resiliency-informed therapist

In choosing a therapist, it is important to find someone who has received training in treatment of traumatic stress and utilizes evidence-supported trauma assessments and treatments. Listings of evidence-supported treatments can be found on the NCTSN website (www.nctsn.org/resources/topics/treatments-that-work/promising-practices), the U.S. National Registry of Evidence-based Programs and Practices (NREPP) developed by the U.S. Substance Abuse Mental Health Services Administration (www.federalregister.gov/documents/2015/07/07/2015-16573/national-registry-of-evidence-based-programs-and-practices*) and the California Evidence-based Clearinghouse for Child Welfare (*www.cebc4cw.org). To locate a trauma therapist, please see: www.istss.org. In the United States, resources to find a therapist include the American Psychological Association's locator guide: https://locator.apa.org/?_ga=2.1130609.1963255459.1582577354-1975622439.1582140597.

For children who have experienced multiple types of traumas and impaired relationships with caregivers, it is important to use a treatment model developed and tested for Complex Trauma and matching the developmental level of the child. Evidence-supported treatment models for Complex Trauma with elementary school-age children and adolescents functioning socially, emotionally, and cognitively, at a 6–12-year-old level, include *Real Life Heroes® (RLH)*, a resiliency-centered treatment model developed by the author of *The Hero's Mask* along with other evidence-supported treatments such as: *Attachment, Regulation and Competence* (ARC), *Integrated Treatment For Complex Trauma* (ITCT), *Trauma Systems Therapy* (TST) and adaptations of Trauma-focused Cognitive Behavioral Therapy (TF-CBT) for Complex Trauma.[2] For children under age 6, please see information on: *Child Parent Psychotherapy*. For group trauma treatment models, please see: *Trauma Affect Regulation: Guide for Education and Therapy (TARGET), STAIR Narrative Therapy,* and *Structured Psychotherapy for Adolescents Responding to Chronic Stress (SPARCS)*. Information on these treatments can be found on the NCTSN, NREPP and CEBC websites listed above and in the resource list in Chapter 6 of this guidebook.

Notes

1 Please see Lieberman, A. & van Horn, P. (2011). *Psychotherapy with Infants and Young Children: Repairing the Effects of Stress and Trauma on Early Attachment.* New York: Guilford for a guide to helping parents rebuild attachments with young children after traumas.

2 Please see Cohen, J.A. Mannarino, A.P., & Deblinger, E. (2017). *Treating Trauma and Traumatic Grief in Children and Adolescents,* 2nd Edn. New York: Guilford for a guide to treatment of traumatic grief.

3. Developing trauma-informed schools and child and family service programs

The Hero's Mask can be used to help schools and child and family service programs to develop projects, treatment programs, and policies that help prevent and ameliorate traumatic stress and build skills and supportive relationships to increase resilience. The book provides an engaging format and resource to:

- Promote activities and dialogues with children that build on family and cultural strengths, normalize trauma reactions, and promote resiliency including the importance of emotionally supportive relationships for every child.
- Model how caregivers, teachers, counselors, and schools can help children in distress to develop the security, perspective, confidence, and skills needed to overcome common challenges in classrooms and schools and to change disruptive behavior into behaviors that promote success and educational achievement.
- Augment social studies curricula with classroom activities using imagery from heroes' stories and supplemented by activities and homework assignments that expand understanding of traumatic stress and building resilience.
- Encourage schools and other community organizations to prevent and manage bullying and to replace fear-driven policies and protocols that can stifle learning with trauma and resiliency-informed policies and protocols.

Psychoeducation on trauma and resilience

Reading *The Hero's Mask* helps normalize trauma reactions and promotes key components for healing and prevention of future traumatic reactions including trauma psychoeducation, emotionally supportive relationships for children with caregivers and teachers, safety from bullying and violence, developing courage as an antidote to fears and working together to prevent and reduce toxic effects of traumatic events.

The 'tough times' experienced by Carrie represent common difficulties experienced by many children and families. The book demonstrates how experiences of multiple types of trauma, even at a moderate level, can strain emotionally supportive relationships in families, lead to parental unavailability, and engender a growing detachment of children from other family members. The book shows how family conflicts can, in turn, lead to greater sensitivity by children to stressors in schools, decreased capacity for focusing attention in school, vulnerability to negative peer influences, decreased school achievement, and behavioral problems.

The Hero's Mask can be used to promote discussions and activities designed to foster recovery and renewal of a family's and community's heritage, values, and resources that have enabled families to persevere and overcome hard times. The book includes references to values Carrie learned from her grandmother and her family that can encourage parents and caregivers sharing with their children family stories of overcoming and strengths in their cultural heritage.

Community and cultural issues that affect children's mental health and success in schools are also addressed in *The Hero's Mask*. References to 'Don't ask, Don't tell, Don't look, Don't see' can be used to discuss how this can help families and communities avoid facing difficult issues; and, at the same time, how this can constrict children's trust in adults to protect them, safety for children to share experiences and children seeking adults' help in making things better. *The Hero's Mask* can be used to model how to break down barriers to communication between children and adults and to promote building on strengths and healing from stressful or traumatic events. *The Hero's Mask* encourages adults to model how they can be the protectors and leaders children and communities need.

Empowering caregivers and strengthening emotionally supportive relationships

The Hero's Mask highlights the importance of caring adults' commitment to their children during 'tough times' and how caregivers can rebuild emotionally supportive relationships that have been strained by traumatic events. Encouraging adults to read the book helps empower caregivers to re-assert vital roles in reestablishing the safety, nurture and guidance children need to develop vital skills and succeed and reinforces how parents and other caregivers provide models for children on how to manage stressful events.

Reading *The Hero's Mask* can encourage children to share their own traumatic experiences after thinking about Carrie's experiences and reactions. To make this successful, it is important for trauma-informed schools and programs to establish referral processes to help children and families who disclose traumatic events or seek help for traumatic stress. This includes access to therapists trained in evidence-supported trauma treatments for PTSD and Complex Trauma.

Therapists in trauma-informed programs can encourage parents and children to read the book together or separately with follow-up discussions with therapists when needed. Reading the book can help adults understand how stressful events and adult reactions contribute to common behavioral problems and engage parents and caregivers' support and involvement in treatment. The story provides a model for how caregivers can help children to develop the security, perspective, confidence, and skills needed to overcome challenges and to replace behavioral problems with behaviors that succeed.

Moving from trauma awareness to trauma-informed action[1]

The Hero's Mask can help schools and programs move *beyond* awareness of how ACES and traumas affect children and families and to develop sustainable trauma-informed policies, procedures, and services. This includes on-going psychoeducation programs for caregivers and training programs for teachers and other school staff, juvenile justice staff, social services staff, courts and security officers. Trauma training programs can be accessed through the National Child Traumatic Stress Network (www.nctsn.org) along with guides to the NCTSN Core Concepts of Childhood Trauma which provide a framework for addressing childhood trauma and adversity. Please see *What is a Trauma-Informed Child and Family Service System* at www.nctsn.org for a guide to components of trauma-informed systems. Evidence-supported programs that have been successful in developing trauma-informed programs include *Attachment, Regulation, Competency* (https://arcframework.org), *Sanctuary* (www.sanctuaryweb. com), and *Trauma Systems Therapy* (www.nctsn.org/interventions/trauma-systems-therapy). For a guide to evaluating development of trauma-informed programs, please see the *Trauma-Informed Organizational Assessment (TIOA): Informational Packet,* also available at www.nctsn.org.

Trauma-informed programs utilize trauma screening and assessment tools and develop treatment and educational plans that reinforce safety, strengthen supportive relationships and help children build skills. Promoting resilience is a critical part of effective treatment programs including promoting resilience for caring adults and service providers experiencing secondary traumatic stress. Trauma-informed programs need to be able to link children and families to evidence-supported treatments and programs that help strengthen or build attachments, increase self and co-regulation skills for managing stressors, and reintegrate traumatic memories.

Note

1 Joseph Benamati (2013). Personal communication.

4. Curriculum guide for educators and use in groups

Teachers can use *The Hero's Mask* to enrich students' understanding of what it feels like to experience traumatic stress, what can lead to increased stress and behavioral problems and how to promote resilience with skill-building and emotional support. The book illustrates how students, teachers and schools can deal with common challenges including setting rules for classroom safety from emotional or physical abuse, managing youths who bully peers, and pressure on teachers and students to achieve on standardized testing. Reading the book can increase children's curiosity about what is happening in their schools, communities and families. Carrie, the main character models perseverance and pushing past boundaries. *The Hero's Mask* highlights what students, teachers, parents, administrators, and community leaders can do to help children and families recover after traumatic events including fostering relationships, courage and creativity and moving beyond implicit or explicit limits that constrict prevention or healing from traumatic stress.

The *Hero's Project* activities described in the book can be linked to mastery of core academic subjects (literature, science, social studies) and educational achievement to generate interest and motivation to learn. These activities can be used to help teachers to develop stronger relationships with children and to create openings to model how adults and children can work together to grow stronger after traumatic events. Classroom and homework activities can be expanded using the suggestions below to promote students' feelings of belonging, curiosity, and sense of competence to manage common stressors.

The Hero's Mask can also be used in therapeutic groups for children to promote understanding and normalization of trauma responses. A group format can be helpful for increasing motivation and support for trying out new behaviors and to reinforce how children are not alone if they have experienced traumatic events.

Suggested use of *The Hero's Mask* is outlined below for use in 4th–6th grade classrooms. This guide can be adapted for use with adolescents or for use in psychotherapeutic groups. For further information, guidelines, tips, and resources for educators on using an understanding of traumatic stress in schools, please see: www.nctsn.org/sites/default/files/assets/pdfs/CTTE_Educators.pdf. The National Child Traumatic Stress Network (NCTSN) has also developed a *Child Trauma Toolkit for Educators* which is available at: www.nctsn.org/resources/audiences/school-personnel/trauma-toolkit. For additional activities on using the hero's metaphor to promote skill development in conjunction with trauma treatment, please see:

Kagan, R. (2004). *Rebuilding Attachments with Traumatized Children*. New York: Routledge;

Kagan, R. (2017). *Real Life Heroes Life Storybook*, 3rd Edn. New York: Routledge; and

Kagan, R. (2017). *Real Life Heroes Toolkit for Treating Traumatic stress in Children and Families*. New York: Routledge.

Themes for discussion elicited by reading *The Hero's Mask*

Courage—Taking risks

Heroes—Attributes, myths, models for skill-building

Coming of age—Figuring out who you are, what matters and what you are willing to fight for

Peer relationships

Inner feelings compared to feelings shown to others

Difficult experiences: Losses of family members you love, parental conflict, parental depression and unavailability for children, bullies

Impact of community problems on families: job losses, economic problems, increased stress, exhaustion

Growing stronger by integrating new skills and relationships after going through 'tough times'

Developing resilience—Emotionally supportive relationships and coping skills

Curriculum connections with core subjects

Language Arts: Writing stories, Vocabulary

Social Studies: Psychology, Trauma, Resilience, Communities, Education

Science: How traumatic stress develops and how common behavioral responses help and hurt, what works to alleviate emotional distress, what can increase emotional distress, what does healing and growth after trauma mean?

Curriculum objectives[1]

After reading *The Hero's Mask* and participating in discussion groups, students will be able to do the following at levels appropriate for their developmental age:

- Identify types of experiences that can lead to traumatic stress and ways trauma impacts the lives of children and adults.
- Describe in simple terms normal reactions to trauma events (behaviors, bodily reactions, thoughts, feelings, social interactions).
- Describe ways that parents, teachers, neighbors, and friends can help prevent traumatic stress, and prevent or reduce shame and stigmatization after traumatic events.
- Recognize bullying and develop and implement ways to prevent or stop abusive behavior by children.
- Describe ways that families, schools, and communities can help children get stronger after traumatic events and ways students can help peers who have experienced traumatic stress.

For more advanced groups:

- Describe what resilience to stressful experiences means and what can be done to promote resilience in children, families, and communities.
- Describe how Carrie's story is similar to the stages of the Hero's Journey[2] outlined by Joseph Campbell and how other stories of heroes follow this sequence of stages.

Before children read the book

Generate curiosity by encouraging children to:

- Read over the Contents and discuss what they expect to happen in the book.
- Provide resource information on traumatic stress and complex trauma, e.g. from NCTSN materials for children and adolescents.
- Collect information on traumatic stress and complex trauma and make these available for caregivers (see references above and in Chapter 2).
- Encourage children to start a personal journal to increase self-reflection and to use writing to share feelings and help express their own feelings, concerns or distress.

Teachers should be aware of students who may be triggered by reminders of loss, family conflicts, emotional abuse, neglect or bullying and enlist help from counseling staff and supervisors to support these students. Discussions and activities can be tailored to prevent over-stimulation about sensitive issues by leaving out specific activities and providing students with options to leave activities and meet with counselors or administrative staff if they feel overly stressed at any time. School counselors can be encouraged to use suggestions in Chapter 5 to help students in evidence-supported counseling to use the book and write stories about 'tough times,' how children and other people made things better after 'tough times,' what children learned about staying safe and making things better from going through 'tough times' and what can be done to prevent future 'tough times' or traumas.

As children read the book

Break children into small groups of three to four to discuss questions (see below).

- Select one child to record group ideas on paper, wall posters, a tablet, or a laptop.
- If time permits, include drawings, collages, or other creative arts to enhance ideas listed.
- Ask each small group to prepare to share these with the class.
- Ideas generated can be shared with other students when completed in print, poster, or digital format. Posters can be mounted on bulletin boards, in halls, or displays in school or community settings.
- Encourage children to share any distress or concerns with people they trust, e.g. parents, grandparents, teachers, counselors, principals, clergy [share how children can meet with school counselors if desired].

Discussion topics

Encourage children to think about each character and discuss in their small groups:

What are characters seeing, feeling, thinking, doing?

What are they looking for?

What is upsetting?

What do they want to happen?

What helps characters?

How do they help each other?

What gets in their way?

What fosters courage to learn what is real?

What fosters courage to get help from others?

What fosters courage to work with others to make things better?

Encourage children to think about heroes and to tackle the same questions addressed in Carrie's class with extra questions and links to grade-level curricula for social studies, science, literature, and writing. Discuss and encourage application of concepts in school, in the community and at home.

Table 4.1   Discussion questions and children's responses illustrated by characters in _The Hero's Mask_

How heroes stay safe: special skills that warn of danger and help heroes escape (Chapters 8–9)

Hearing
Sight
Smell
Touch
Taste
Balance
Concentration
Speed
Strength
Know who they can go to for help, anywhere they are, any time of day or night
Get help when they need it

Lessons from heroes (Chapter 9)

No one is perfect, not even great heroes.
Everybody makes mistakes.
Heroes admit when they are wrong.
Senses and skills are not enough, you need the courage to do something.
Learn from the past but don't get stuck in the past.
Make things better.
It's okay to be scared.
Everyone gets scared. Don't let it stop you from seeing what is happening and doing something to make things better.
Everybody gets scared, so don't be ashamed about being afraid.
Fear is like energy.
We can use fear to grow our own power, the power to do what we need to do.

Doing something is better than being stuck.

Take little steps, one step at a time, and even big jobs get done!

Secrets of heroes to stay safe (Chapter 12)

Parents and other caring adults who keep you safe and help you learn how to stay safe.

Open your eyes and ears (and nose) to find out if it's safe.

Get help from friends, getting help makes it easier to explore, to learn, to be brave, to get away from danger and to become safe again.

Secrets of heroes to keep moving in 'tough times'[3] (Chapter 19)

The antidote to fear is action.

Action requires courage.

The secret to courage is purpose.

Purpose comes from knowing where you want to go, what you need to do, and that doing it makes all the difference.

And, once you know what you need to do, then you can look at fear in other ways.

Fear can be the alarm that says 'get ready.'

Fear can give us the energy to move, to fight, to escape, and to make things better.

Discussion questions and activities for selected chapters and topics

Educators can select additional assignment ideas from the list below and develop their own projects to match their students and the community's cultural heritage.

Chapters 3–4: How can schools and classrooms encourage learning?

Think about how our school encourages learning.

- What helps students learn?
- What gets in the way?
- What would you do if you were a teacher or principal to help students learn?
- Are there other ways students can show what they have learned besides taking tests? How can tests help? How do we use tests? What else could help show learning?

Chapter 7: How can we recognize heroes and bullies?

Think of someone who you think acted as a hero.

- What special qualities does your hero show?
- What special skills do they use?
- Who helped them learn these skills and become a hero?
- What was one heroic thing your hero did?

Think of someone who you think acted like a bully.

- How do you recognize bullying? [Discussion points: different forms of bullying, does bullying have to be physical?]
- If someone acts like a bully and makes other children feel bad, how do you think that helps the person acting like a bully? What does this say about how they see themselves?
- Can adults be bullies to each other? Can adults be bullies to children?
- What stops bullies? [Discussion points: getting help from teachers, administrators, other children, parents, neighbors; using your skills to stay strong, giving bullies messages to stop, working together to present a united front against bullying in all forms.]
- What rules does the class and school already have to stop bullies?
- Would any other rules help?
- What can each student do to help someone who is bullied? What can teachers do? School administrators? Parents? Police? Judges?

Extra project

The Hero's Mask can be incorporated into anti-bullying programs in schools. Issues to be addressed include discussion questions above and identifying responsibilities (what, when, how) for: administrators, teachers, clergy, police, state, city (or town) government leaders, parents, grandparents, aunts, uncles, older siblings and children.

Chapter 8: What helps heroes succeed and what can we learn about heroes?

Think of someone who made their country, their state or province, or their city or village better, someone you think of as a hero, someone you would like to learn more about. Then, use the library, computer and other resources to learn more about what this hero did, what helped them overcome challenges, and how she/he made things better.

- What helped them overcome the hardships and 'tough times' they faced?
- What special skills or relationships helped them to succeed?
- What kept them going when they faced hard times or when people told them they couldn't 'do it' or that they should just stop and quit before something bad happened?

Chapter 9: What can heroes teach us about safety, skills, and getting past 'tough times'?

Think of the heroes you admire.

- What helped to keep your heroes safe?
- What are some other special skills heroes learn?
- Is it okay for heroes to ask for help?
- Who could help you learn skills you need to stay safe?

Think about what your own 'Secrets of Staying Safe' would be.

- Would you use your senses?
- Would you get help? How?

- Write out your own 'Secrets of Staying Safe.'
- Who could help you follow your 'Secrets of Staying Safe' and make them work?
- Practice your hero skills today, tonight, and every day this week.
- Then, write a second page about how you used your senses to protect yourself and other people.

Think about lessons you have learned from heroes.

- Do heroes have to be perfect? Are heroes usually perfect? [Discussion point: Is it possible to be perfect?]
- Do heroes work alone? [Discussion point: discuss the myth of the solitary hero and contrast with how soldiers, sports teams, and scientists working on projects describe the importance of working together, looking out for each other, and teamwork.]
- Do heroes have secret powers? [Discussion points: Use examples of normal people who find themselves in a difficult situation and muster the courage to help others, even if it means taking risks for themselves. Can we find special strengths within ourselves, our families or our communities?]
- Can mistakes help us?

Homework assignment

Ask someone in your family about their favorite hero. You can ask a parent, a grandparent, a brother, a sister, a cousin, or even a very close family friend.

- Who is their favorite hero?
- How did this hero use his/her senses to warn them of danger?
- What were some of the special skills this hero used to sense danger and help themselves and other people?
- Who helped this hero develop their special skills?
- What were some of the things this hero did to make things better for other people?
- Who helped this hero help other people?
- What is one lesson we can learn from this hero?

Chapters 11–12: What lessons can we learn from animals to help us know how to escape from 'tough times' and make things better?

Think about the frog experiment and what it teaches us.

- What would it take to warn the frog to escape?
- What warning systems could you put in place to protect a frog from the water getting too hot?

Think about what makes a frog special.

- What special abilities does it have?
- How does it use its tongue, nose, legs, skin?
- What can the frog do to escape danger?

Homework assignment

Learn more about the favorite hero of someone in your family or a close family friend.

- What did this hero watch out for as a signal that she/he needed to do something?
- What did this hero do to escape from dangers and to make things better?
- How did this hero get help from other people?
- How did this hero help other people?
- What kept this hero going when things got tough?

Think about the experiment with the little rats.

- What did the cat hair mean to the rats?
- How did their reaction help them?
- What could help the rats feel safe after the cat hair was put into their cage?
- What can we learn from this experiment to help children who experience dangerous people or risks of severe harm?
- What does PTSD mean?
- What are some of the signs of PTSD?
- Did the little rats show signs of PTSD?
- What other ways could scientists learn about how animals cope with hard times or traumas?

Further homework assignments

Find a story from books or movies about heroes and write about the lessons that one of the heroes learned from something he/she was afraid of.

- What traumatic experiences does your hero go through?
- What helps your hero get through 'tough times'?
- How does your hero help other people?
- What risks does your hero take to help others?
- Does the hero you picked disguise their identity in any way, for example by wearing a mask, different clothes, or changing their hair color or how they talk or act?
- Does hiding your identity (who you really are) help heroes? How?
- Does hiding your feelings sometimes help?
- Can hiding your feelings get in the way sometimes?
- Think about your hero and explain what these experiences and skills meant for your hero: traumas, survival skills, mentors, healing, becoming stronger and stronger to face new 'tough times.' What happened to your hero? How did they show skills? Who and what helped them?
- For advanced students: What is resilience? How does your hero show resilience?

Advanced project

Learn about parts of the brain involved in memory and developing skills to keep safe from harm. How are these parts of the brain affected by experiencing a trauma? What happens when a boy, girl, man, or woman experiences multiple traumas over many years and believes they are still unsafe?[4] Write about an example of someone who went through a trauma and found a way to recover? What helped?

Chapter 13: What are some types of 'tough times' that can lead to severe stress, intense fears, and trauma reactions?

Think of the 'tough times' Carrie experienced in her family.

- What are some problems that feel like traumas?
- Can losing jobs be a threat to a family? Can losing a parent's job be like the cat hair in the experiment with the little rats?
- Do you know anyone whose parents lost a job?
- Do you know anyone who goes to bed hungry?
- What could other people do to help them?
- Is there anything a class could do to help children in families who have lost jobs?
- Can losing a grandparent be traumatic?
- Can losing a parent be traumatic?
- Can living with a parent who spends a lot of his/her time crying or sleeping in bed and appears tired and angry most of the time be traumatic for children?
- Can experiencing parents fight with words be traumatic for children?
- Can experiencing parents fight in a way that causes bodily harm be traumatic for children?
- What happens to a child or adult when stressful or traumatic events keep happening over and over?
- What happens when many different types of stressful or traumatic events keep happening, for instance the death of a parent, physical abuse and bullying at school? Is that different for a child than just experiencing one type of trauma?

Feelings and worries have been described as being like waves rolling onto a beach and then rolling out again, one wave after another.[5] They can look big or small, but they all flow onto the shore and then slip back out to sea. In the same way, feelings like fears or worries can be seen as flowing in and then flowing away, one after another.

- Do you think feelings are like waves that come and go?
- What else do feelings remind you of? [Discussion points: consider other images that are like feelings, e.g. cars passing below a city apartment building or along a highway, leaves floating down a stream, a train passing by, car by car.]
- Do you think the same is true for thoughts, like worries, that they too can come crashing in but then flow out to be replaced by another thought or worry, one after another?
- Does it help to know that feelings and thoughts come and go for everybody, that what you may be feeling right now, however strong it is, will pass on and that another feeling or thought will come, and then another?

- Does it help to know that you can change the feelings and thoughts you have? [Discussion points: Use yoga moves, slow breathing, stretching, smiling, laughing to experiment with changing our feelings.]

Imagine sitting high on a bluff far, far above a beach, higher than any wave could reach, and looking at waves[6] coming in from ocean.

- If a large wave came, would it feel scary or dangerous for you? If so, would it help to get even higher or further away?
- Can waves help people?
- How do surfers use waves?
- Can waves help create energy like electricity to light up our homes?
- What helps us to enjoy a beach safely? [Discussion Points: lifeguards, weather forecasts, ocean forecasts, buddies, parents.]

Extra project

How can we use the same ways we stay safe on a beach to keep us safe in other places? Write out a plan for one place children and parents might go, for example, hiking in the mountains, swimming in a lake, taking a train to another city, taking the subway downtown, going to a large shopping mall, visiting a city in another country, going to a new school. What can help children stay safe in that place?

Chapter 15: What helps children get through tough times?

Think of childhood games like *Ring Around the Rosie.*

- How did it help children?
- What songs or games do children sing now that helps them get through 'tough times' in their lives?
- Can stories of heroes help children get through hard times? How?
- What could help little children like Carrie's brother?

Extra project

What helps you get through hard times? Write out ways that help including things you can do by yourself, with your family, and with friends.

Chapter 16: How can reminders of traumas lead to feeling like you are re-living a terrible experience?

Think about what led up to Carrie's fight in the cafeteria.

- What do you think led up to her getting into a fight?
- How did broken glass work as a reminder? Blood? Words like 'crazy'?
- What else, besides sounds, can be a reminder of traumatic experiences? [Discussion points: smells, looks on

people's faces, tone of voice, words used, threats, violence, time of day, time of year, activities at home or school, interactions.]

- Did the cafeteria aide or security officer know what was really happening?
- What else could the cafeteria aide and security officer have done to help?
- What could have helped Carrie avoid getting into trouble?

Think about what happened to Carrie after the fight.

- If you were the principal and you heard what happened in the cafeteria, what would you want to find out?
- How would you try to prevent bullying?
- How would you try to help children who have been hurt before at home or in school from being hurt again or getting into trouble?
- How can writing a story of a really bad time help?
- Does it help to share the story? With whom?
- Is there anyone you wouldn't you want to share your story with to keep yourself and others safe? If so, how can you keep your stories safe?
- Does it help to include a plan for making things better and preventing future bad times in your stories, or, if the bad times can't be prevented, to make them less difficult?
- What else helps?

Chapter 18: How do you think masks can help?

Think about what Carrie learned about masks.

- Why do heroes wear masks?
- What heroes in books or movies do you know who wore masks?
- Do you think hiding or faking feelings is like a mask?
- What heroes in books or movies hid their feelings?
- What other things do people do to hide what they are thinking or feeling?
- Does it help people sometimes to hide their feelings? Is it necessary?

Homework assignment

Write about how a hero you admire from books or movies uses a mask or another way to hide their feelings. How does it help them to make things better? How do they know who they can trust to share their real feelings and thoughts? What lessons can we learn from this hero to know when we can share our real feelings?

Extra project

Think of Carrie's nightmare of children being forced to 'Don't ask. Don't tell. Don't hear. Don't see' and the experiment with the frog.

- What happens if you 'don't ask or don't tell, don't hear or don't see'?
- Can this be helpful in some ways?
- Can it be harmful in some ways?
- Write about how our beliefs can shape what we say, think and do.

Chapters 19–22: What helps children and adults be brave enough to take risks to make things better?

Think about what helped heroes you admire.

- What helps heroes in books and movies be brave? [Discussion points: family, mentors, friends, feeling a strong need to make things better after something bad happened, caring about someone.]
- Did these heroes feel at any time that they did not want to do what was needed to make things better or that they couldn't do anything to help?
- Do real heroes feel afraid sometimes?
- What helps real people, children and adults, be brave? [Discussion points: support from other people, mentors, friends, keeping an important goal in mind, feeling like they can make a difference.]
- Can heroes use their fear to help them keep going? [Discussion point: how fear is natural and a source of energy needed to take action and make things better.]
- What stories do you know of real people in your family who took risks to help others and make things better?
- What stories do you know of real people in your community (town, city) or this country who took risks to help others and make things better? [Discussion points: Heroes can be boys, girls, women, men, all cultural groups, from farms or cities, all over the world.]
- What makes it harder to have the courage to make things better?
- What makes it easier?
- Does it help for heroes to share what they learned with other people?

Homework assignment

Write a story of someone who overcame great hardships or who took risks to make things better for other people. How did they deal with fears? Who helped them learn skills to succeed? Who helped them make things better? What did they learn from struggling to make things better? Did they share what they learned with anyone?

Chapters 20–21: What helps children and adults keep going when things get tough?

Think about Carrie at the school board meeting.

- What lessons from her family and her own experience helped her to speak up?
- What did the school board president do to make Carrie feel less confident?
- How did it help the school board president to point out Carrie's problems at school? Is this fair?
- What helps children or adults keep going when someone points out past problems or blames them for causing trouble? [Discussion points: What can we do to can remind ourselves of our strengths, our goals,

people who care enough to help us? How can we understand what other people are doing including people who act in abusive ways and how can we use that understanding to stay strong?]

- If you feel you have been falsely blamed for something, how can you make things better? What can other people (parents, teachers, other students) do to help?
- If you feel you have done something wrong in the past, how can you make things better? [Discussion points: How do you make up for hurting someone in your family or religion? Is it important to apologize? Is it important to try to make up for what did you did wrong? How can this be done?]
- How did having Carrie's friends and their parents at the school board meeting help Carrie?
- How did Carrie's mother help? How did thinking of what Carrie's grandmother would have done help Carrie's mother?
- Who else could have helped Carrie if her mother didn't come to the meeting? [Discussion points: Could Principal Pratt have helped? Carrie's friends' parents? Carrie's friends? Ms. Kramer? Carrie's uncle?]
- If a child's own mother or father can't or won't help, who else could help a child?
- How do families, communities, religions, and cultures teach lessons of heroes and pass them along from one generation to another?

Extra homework assignments

Think about this statement:

'It takes action to free ourselves from living in fear.

Action requires energy to move.

We can get energy by using our fears. Everyone has fears. We feel fear in our bodies. Fears warn us to be ready. Fears can energize us to move. We can use fears as energy to move forwards or lose ourselves in the grip of our fears. Accepting and using our fears makes us stronger.

Action also requires courage.

The secret to courage is purpose. It means finding out what you need to do to make things better. And, it means believing with all your heart that something you can do can make a difference.

But action alone does not make a real hero.

Action for heroes means doing something to make things better and doing it together with other people who help each other. Action for heroes means helping others and getting help for ourselves.'[7]

Discuss and add creative arts for imagery, rhythm, tonality, or movement to highlight responses:

- What do you think helps people avoid becoming trapped in fear?
- What would help someone who was trapped?

- Can fears or terror be like something that makes you feel sick?
- Can fears or terror work like a sort of poison?
- How do antidotes work for poison?
- Does 'action' work like an antidote to feeling trapped in fear?
- Is there a way to help people develop the courage to do something when they are afraid?
- What helps you do something when things are scary or hard?
- Why is it important to get help for ourselves as well as helping others?
- What would you tell another boy or girl who you believed was feeling like they were trapped or stuck with a lot of fear and having trouble escaping?
- Write what you would tell this child as a message.

Homework assignment

Share a time when someone helped you feel better after a 'tough time' or you helped someone else. What helped? What was the 'antidote' to the 'tough time,' something that helped take away the distress and make things better?

After children read the book

- Encourage children in groups to discuss what are 'tough times.'
    What helps people get through them?
    What makes us feel like we are stuck in 'tough times'? What does that feel like?
    What helps us cope? [Discussion points: How can parents, siblings, aunts, uncles and other family members help? How can friends, neighbors, teachers, school administrators, clergy, mentors and other caring adults help?]
    How can we develop greater skills to cope with 'tough times'?
    What makes stress become traumatic?
    What helps us prevent or reduce traumatic stress? [Discussion points: How does curiosity help prevent and reduce traumatic stress? How can supportive relationships help prevent or reduce traumatic stress?]
    How does curiosity and learning help prevent feeling trapped?
    Are there typical things that happen to heroes?
    Are there typical stages in stories about heroes? [Discussion points: use Joseph Campbell's concepts about the 'Hero's Journey' with age-appropriate references to parts of popular stories and movies, e.g. *Star Wars*, *Harry Potter*, The *Wizard of Oz*.]
- Write your own story using Campbell's stages. [Discussion points: For older children, Campbell's 12 stages can be used with illustrations from contemporary movies or books ('Ordinary World, Call to Adventure, Refusal of The Call, Meeting the Mentor, Crossing the Threshold, Tests, Allies, Enemies, Approach to Inmost Cave, Ordeal, Reward (Seizing the Sword), the Road Back, Resurrection, Return with Elixir'). For younger children, Campbell's stages can be simplified, or his broad outline used: 'Departure, Initiation, Return.'] Children can be encouraged to write a three-chapter story with a beginning, middle and end with the last chapter highlighting how characters made things better.

- Share concerns or any feelings of distress with someone you trust. [Share how children can meet with school counselors if desired, in addition to parents, relatives, teachers, mentors, clergy and other caring adults they feel safe with.]

Advanced homework assignments

Write your own hero story using the stages discussed based on Joseph Campbell. [Discussion points: Introduce story structures often used in fiction books: introduction, challenges, twist, climax, or movies using adaptations of Campbell's stages. Ask students to identify these in their stories.]

In the book, Ms. Kramer says she was inspired by Albert Einstein. Encourage students to learn about what shaped his life. What 'tough times' did he have to manage? Encourage students to think about what Einstein meant and share their own thoughts about famous quotes from Einstein:

'Imagination is more important than knowledge.'

'In the middle of difficulty lies opportunity.'

[Discussion points: Do you think these are true? How can you use them in your own life? Who inspires you? What have you learned from them? What other quotes inspire you?]

Notes

1 Objectives can be modified to match time available and students' level of development.
2 Campbell, J. (1968). *The Hero with a Thousand Faces*. Princeton, NJ: Princeton University Press.
3 Adapted from Kagan, R. (2017). *Real Life Heroes Life Storybook*, 3rd Edn. New York: Routledge.
4 For a resource, please see: Spinazzola, J., Habib, M., Blaustein, M., Knoverek, A., Kisiel, C., Stolbach, B., Abramovitz, R., Kagan, R., Lanktree, C., and Maze, J. (2017). *What is Complex Trauma? A Resource Guide for Youth and Those Who Care About Them*. Los Angeles, CA, and Durham, NC: National Center for Child Traumatic Stress (available at www.nctsn.org).
5 Marra, T. (2004). *Depressed and Anxious: The Dialectical Behavior Therapy Workbook for Overcoming Depression and Anxiety*. Oakland, CA: New Harbinger Press.
6 Ibid.
7 Kagan, R. (2017a). *The Real Life Heroes Life Storybook*, 3rd Edn. New York: Routledge, p. 243.

5. Use by psychotherapists and counselors

Engagement

Trauma therapists often cite engagement and sustaining engagement as the greatest challenges in trauma treatment, especially for Complex Trauma. *The Hero's Mask* promotes engagement by normalizing common experiences and reactions in a format that accentuates hope and children's and parents' natural yearning to make things better. The book can be especially helpful to engage children and families with traumatic grief and to strengthen parent-child relationships that have become frayed after multiple traumas in families, schools and communities. Encouraging children and their parents or caregivers to read the book can elicit feelings of caring and new ways to help troubled and troubling children, which can, in turn, lead to renewed hope and commitments by caring adults to help the children they love.

The Hero's Mask helps empower parents and caregivers by showing how trauma impacts children and families *and* how parents and other caring adults can help their children and themselves. The book can be used to support essential components in trauma treatments including development of safe, emotionally supportive relationships, self- and co-regulation skill-building, overcoming shame, re-integration of traumatic memories, and building a stronger sense of competence and identity for children, families and communities. As with any treatment intervention, use of *The Hero's Mask* should follow a comprehensive assessment and safety plans including an assessment of children's capacity to manage stress with the help of safe parents and caregivers.

Increasing safety to share

Therapists and counselors can utilize Carrie and her family's experiences as models for:

- Recognizing traumatic stress reactions and how avoidance, denial, and conflict can cover up underlying feelings of distress or shame, e.g. Carrie feeling she didn't do enough to keep her father from leaving.
- Identifying triggers to traumatic reactions, e.g. broken glass for Carrie.
- Identifying what is needed to help children and caregivers in a family become safe enough to share feelings.
- Learning from heroes in children's families, communities, and from their cultural heritage and how to apply what is learned to problems facing a child or family in the present time, e.g. modeling by Carrie's grandmother and how that inspired Carrie's mother.

- Learning with whom a child can safely share trauma experiences.
- Developing safety plans to prevent and reduce traumatic stress reactions including safety signals for use in school and at home, e.g. the 'C code' used by Carrie and her friends.
- Enhancing children's curiosity and exploration of ways to make their lives better, e.g. writing out what happened and what could make things better.
- Identifying talents and enhancing skills in children that can help them stay modulated when stressed, e.g. soccer for Carrie.
- Encouraging writing stories and therapeutic story-telling[1] that can help children 'move through' traumas to a safe ending where they feel emotionally connected to other people.

Carrie's story portrays common efforts by children and adults to suppress or avoid facing traumas in order to help themselves cope with overwhelming distress. Therapists can encourage children and caregivers to identify what was most disturbing for Carrie, how fears kept her from grieving losses of her father and grandmother, how reminders of traumas (triggers) led to dysregulated behavior, e.g. her legs kicking wildly or the cafeteria fight, and how emotionally supportive relationships with friends, her new teacher, and her family helped her to become stronger and able to do what she believed she needed to do to help her school. Before doing this, it would be important, as with any treatment intervention, to begin with a comprehensive assessment and any necessary safety plans including an assessment of children's capacity to manage stress with the help of parents and caregivers.

Secrets of heroes: helping others and getting help for oneself

Learning about heroes provides a segue for looking at what can help children who have experienced multiple losses and feel unable to overcome feelings of regret or shame. Carrie, her mother, her friends, her new teacher, and her school principal provide models for how ordinary people can find ways to make things better in 'tough times,' including for Carrie and her mother feeling they have hurt people they loved. Regret, guilt and shame are primary factors in traumatic stress and interfere with children's, families' and communities' capacity to grieve losses and become stronger together after re-integrating traumatic experiences. Healing includes developing renewed pride in one's abilities, one's family and heritage and often rebuilding (or rebuilding) relationships that have become torn or strained.

Seeking help and helping others is emphasized throughout the book as primary lessons from people who become real life heroes. This helps children, families and communities move beyond images of a mythical solitary hero or beliefs that each child or parent must face challenges alone. In treatment, modeling by heroes can be used to encourage children to get help from trustworthy family members, teachers, mentors, clergy and other caring adults and to use this help to develop skills and supportive networks for making things better and protecting against repeated traumas. Modeling by heroes can also be used to encourage children to share what they have learned and done to make things better to help others facing similar 'tough times.' This can include writing a message to help another child who is facing some of the same problems as the child in treatment.

Healing from traumatic stress

The Hero's Mask can be used to normalize experiences of loss and to highlight the importance of strengthening or rebuilding emotionally supportive relationships to help children and parents/caregivers grieve after deaths or other losses. The book illustrates how parent-child relationships can become strained or impaired following multiple stressful events and how detachment and parental unavailability contribute to risks for children and families. In the book, Carrie yearns to return to the loving relationships with her parents and grandmother she remembers before 'tough times' and deaths impacted her family. She is inspired by her new teacher's lessons about heroes that include increasing self and co-regulation skills and writing out experiences in simple stories. Carrie is also supported by her friends and memories of caring from her parents. Carrie's mother musters the courage and strength to re-connect with Carrie, building on the inspiration of her own mother.

Many parents and caregivers are not aware of how distressed their children have become after deaths or other losses of primary relationships, and therapists, as well as parents/caregivers, may be unaware of traumas children have experienced including feelings of shame over what children feel they did that hurt others. Highly stressed parents and caregivers may be focused on surviving each day and continuing to provide essentials for their children, a roof over their heads, food to eat, warm clothes for winter and basic safety. *The Hero's Mask* promotes respect for what parents and caregivers have done and can be used in therapy to encourage parents and caregivers to share their lessons from family members on overcoming poverty, racism, persecution, war or disasters. Reading *The Hero's Mask* promotes empowering parents and other caregivers as essential protectors and guides for children and strengthening children's ties to their cultural heritage. Increasing parent/caregiver attunement with children helps restore safety for family members to share after 'tough times.' As safety and stability increases, children and caregivers typically disclose or validate suspected traumas to family members, therapists and other people they feel they can trust, making it possible to utilize treatment protocols for desensitization and re-integration of traumas, e.g. Trauma-Focused Cognitive Behavioral Therapy (TF-CBT)[2] or Eye Movement Desensitization and Reprocessing (EMDR).[3]

To promote healing from traumatic stress with therapeutic stories, it is helpful for therapists to:

• Accentuate how children and caregivers can feel safe in the present time, that traumas were finite points of time in the past and that children, parents/caregivers and therapists can find ways for family members to be safe in the future, building on their caring for each other.
• Keep the focus in stories on relational healing. This includes being aware of how parents/caregivers and other family members are managing their own feelings of stress and adjusting interventions to boost parents, caregivers, and other family members capacity to support children sharing stories and becoming stronger. It also means being aware of each child's level of fear of losing their primary parents or caregiver's love.[4]
• Structure sessions and interventions so that children experience that caring adults can tolerate children's affective experiences related to traumatic memories[5] and will continue to love, protect and guide children.[6]

Children who have experienced neglect, abuse or abandonment

Children reading the book may have experienced neglect or abandonment, parental unavailability due to their own distress or economic, emotional, physical, alcohol, drug, or emotional struggles, or parents and other family members who reject or abuse their children. Children may also have been exposed to neglect, abuse and abandonment through the experiences of peers, in news reports, in books, in movies and through social media. Repeated experiences of neglect, abuse or abandonment may reinforce beliefs that parents and other adults really don't care and can't be trusted. Children with these experiences may see the book's ending as something they yearn for but at the same time feel is 'too good to be true.'

The Epilogue was designed to elicit hope and promote development of realistic alternatives for children who continue to experience neglect, parental unavailability or abandonment or doubt that adults can come through and help. Carrie's story can be used to open up and address a child's own experiences staying within the child's 'window of tolerance'[7] for stress. Carrie's yearning for caring and experiences of support can be used to promote work to search for, identify and build emotionally supportive relationships for children with someone who can be trusted and to broaden this search beyond parents and primary caregivers to extended family members, mentors, clergy, teachers, neighbors, and other concerned and safe adults. With increased emotional support from safe caring adults, therapists can help children to accept and grieve losses of love and caring from a parent or relative who died or is not able or willing to re-build an emotionally supportive relationship with a child.

Therapists can use the Epilogue to encourage children to write another ending for the book that would help Carrie, and children like Carrie, to manage, even if their moms or dads can't do what Carrie's mother in the story does. If appropriate, children can be asked to go back to Chapter 21 and imagine Carrie sitting on the stage, feeling like she had lost her father, feeling uncared for by her mother, and being criticized by Ms. Thurman. Who could have helped her? Who cared enough to do something? Who was strong enough to tell the truth?

With support from strengthened (or new) relationships, children can also be helped to understand what happened to parents or previous caregivers who became unable to continue caring for children. Learning about what happened to previous caregivers can help therapists and new caregivers to build and test safety plans for children who fear breakdowns and losses of new relationships. For more information on rebuilding trust after relational traumas, please see resources listed in Chapter 6 including: *Rebuilding Attachments with Traumatized Children* (Kagan, 2004), and treatment programs for Complex Trauma listed in the references below including: *Treating Traumatic Stress in Children and Adolescents: How to Foster Resilience Through Attachment, Self-Regulation, and Competency* (Blaustein, & Kinniburgh, 2019), *Real Life Heroes Life Storybook,* 3rd Edn (Kagan, 2017a), *Real Life Heroes Toolkit for Treating Traumatic Stress in Children and Families*, 2nd Edn (Kagan, 2017b), and *Treating Complex Trauma in Children and Their Families: An Integrative Approach* (Lanktree & Briere, 2016).

Evidence-supported treatments

Use of evidence-supported trauma assessments and treatments is recommended in conjunction with this book. Listings of evidence-supported treatments can be found on the NCTSN website (www.nctsn.org/resources/topics/treatments-that-work/promising-practices), the U.S. National Registry of Evidence-based Programs and Practices (NREPP) developed by the U.S. Substance Abuse Mental Health Services Administration (www.federalregister.gov/documents/2015/07/07/2015-16573/national-registry-of-evidence-based-programs-and-practices) and the California Evidence-based Clearinghouse for Child Welfare (www.cebc4cw.org).

For children who have experienced multiple types of traumas including interpersonal traumas, impaired relationships with caregivers, and demonstrate dysregulation, it is important to use a treatment model developed and tested for Complex Trauma. Treatment models also need to be matched to the developmental level of the child. *The Hero's Mask* can be used with many evidence-supported treatments for Complex PTSD for this age group including: *Attachment, Regulation and Competence* (Blaustein, & Kinniburgh, 2019), *Integrated Treatment For Complex Trauma* (Lanktree, & Briere, 2016), *Real Life Heroes®* (Kagan, 2004, 2017a, 2017b), *Trauma Systems Therapy* (Ellis, Saxe, & Brown, 2015) and adaptations of TF-CBT for Complex Trauma (e.g. Kliethermes, Nanney, Cohen, & Mannarino, 2013). Information on these treatments can be found on the NCTSN and NREPP websites listed above and in the resource list below. The resource list also includes treatment models for older youths and preschool children and group treatment models for Complex Trauma including: *Structured Psychotherapy for Adolescents Responding to Chronic Stress (SPARCS)* (DeRosa, Habib, Pelcovitz, et al., 2006; Habib, Labruna, & Newman, 2013), *STAIR Narrative Therapy (Cloitre et al., 2020)*, and *Trauma Affect Regulation: Guide for Education and Therapy (TARGET)* (Ford, & Russo, 2006).

Real Life Heroes® (RLH) utilizes the 'hero's journey' as a framework for resiliency-centered treatment for elementary school-age children and adolescents with traumatic stress functioning socially, emotionally, and cognitively at a 6–12-year-old level. *RLH* focuses on 'relational healing for relational trauma' (Kagan, 2017b) and four core components for treatment of traumatic stress and Complex PTSD: Relationships, Emotional Self and Co-Regulation, Action Cycles (child-parent interactive behavior patterns) and Life Story Integration. The *Real Life Heroes Toolkit for Treating Traumatic stress in Children and Families* and the *Real Life Heroes Life Storybook* can be used in conjunction with *The Hero's Mask* to inspire courage and to engage and sustain children's and parents/caregivers' work on recommended 'best practice' components for treatment of Complex PTSD (Cook, et al., 2003; Ford, & Cloitre, 2009). The *Real Life Heroes Toolkit* includes resources for complex trauma treatment from assessment to service planning, session structure, evaluation and fidelity measures along with creative arts and movement activities for individual, family and group sessions.

Notes

1 For more information on use of therapeutic storytelling, please see: Kagan, R. (2004). *Rebuilding Attachments with Traumatic Stress*. New York: Routledge; and Kagan, R. (2017). *Real Life Heroes Toolkit for Treating Traumatic Stress in Children*, 2nd Edn. New York: Routledge.

2 Cohen, J., A. Mannarino, A.P., & Deblinger, E. (2017). *Treating Trauma and Traumatic Grief in Children and Adolescents*, 2nd Edn. New York: Guilford.

3 Shapiro, F. (2017). *Eye Movement Desensitization and Reprocessing (EMDR) Therapy, Third Edition: Basic Principles, Protocols, and Procedures*, 3rd Edn. New York: Guilford.

4 Lieberman, A.F., & Van Horn, P. (2005). *"Don't hit my mommy!": A Manual for Child-Parent Psychotherapy with Young Witnesses of Family Violence*. Washington, DC: Zero to Three Press.

5 Lieberman, A. (2011). *Developing the Trauma Narrative: Two Evidence-Based Models*. NCTSN All-Network Conference, Baltimore, Maryland (March 3, 2011).

6 Please see the Kagan, R. (2017). *Real Life Heroes Toolkit for Treating Traumatic Stress in Children*, 2nd Edn. New York: Routledge for a guide to use of life story work to promote healing from traumatic stress and Complex Trauma.

7 See Siegel, D.J., & Bryson, T.P. (2014). *No-Drama Discipline: The Whole-Brain Way to Calm the Chaos and Nurture Your Child's Developing Mind*. New York: Bantam.

6. Resources for trauma treatment and research on traumatic grief

Amos, A., Cunningham, A., & Webber, A. (2019). *Therapeutic Story Start-Ups; Stories, Scenes and Characters to Help Children Explore Their Feelings*. London: Routledge.

Becker-Weidman, A., Ehrmann, L., & LeBow, D. (2012). *The Attachment Therapy Companion*. New York: Norton.

Becker-Weidman, A., & Hughes, D. (2008). Dyadic developmental psychotherapy: An evidence-based treatment for children with complex trauma and disorders of attachment. *Child and Family Social Work*, *13*(3), 329–337.

Blaustein, M., & Kinniburgh, K. (2019). *Treating Traumatic Stress in Children and Adolescents: How to Foster Resilience Through Attachment, Self-Regulation, and Competency*, 2nd Edn. New York: Guilford.

Briere, J. (2019). *Treating Risky and Compulsive Behavior in Trauma Survivors*. New York: Guilford.

Briere, J., & Lanktree, C. (2013). *Integrative treatment of complex trauma for adolescents (ITCT-A): A guide for treatment of multiply-traumatized youth,* 2nd Edn. University of Southern California-Adolescent Trauma Training Center, National Child Traumatic Stress Network, U.S. Department of Substance Abuse and Mental Health services Administration.

Briere, J., & Scott, C. (2014). *Principles of Trauma Therapy. Thousand Oaks, CA*: Sage.

Brohl, K. (2017). *Working with Traumatized Children: A Handbook for Healing*, 3rd Edn. Washington, DC: CWLA Press.

Brom, D., Pat-Horenczyk, R., & Ford, J. (2009). *Treating Traumatized Children: Risk, Resilience and Recovery*. New York: Routledge.

Brooks, R. (1994). Children at risk: Fostering resilience and hope. *American Journal of Orthopsychiatry*, *64*, 545–553.

Child Welfare League of America, www.cwla.org/pubs.

Cloitre, M., Courtois, C.A., Charuvastra, A., Carapezza, R., Stolbach, B.C., & Green, B.L. (2011). Treatment of complex PTSD: Results of the ISTSS expert clinician survey on best practices. *Journal of Traumatic Stress*, *24*, 615–627.

Cloitre, M., Cohen, L.R., Ortigo, K.M., Jackson, O., & Koenen, K.C. (2020). *Treating Survivors of Childhood Abuse and Interpersonal Trauma: STAIR Narrative Therapy*, 2nd Edn. New York: Guilford.

Cognitive Behavioral Intervention for Trauma in Schools. See: https://cbitsprogram.org/.

Cohen, J.A. Mannarino, A.P., & Deblinger, E. (2017). *Treating Trauma and Traumatic Grief in Children and Adolescents*, 2nd Edn. New York: Guilford.

Cook, A., Blaustein, M., Spinazzola, J., & van der Kolk, B. (Eds) (2003). *Complex Trauma in Children and Adolescents*. National Child Traumatic Stress Network. www.NCTSNet.org.

Cook, A., Spinazzola, J., Ford, J., Lanktree, C., Blaustein, M., Cloitre, M., DeRosa, R., Hubbard, R., Kagan, R., Liautaud, J., Mallah, K., Olafson, E., & van der Kolk, B. (2005). Complex trauma in children and adolescents. *Psychiatric Annals*, *35*(5), 390–400.

DeRosa, R., Habib, M., & Pelcovitz, D. (2006). *Structured Psychotherapy for Adolescents Responding to Chronic Stress*. Los Angeles, CA: National Child Traumatic Stress Network.

Ellis, B.H., Saxe, G.N., & Brown, A. (2015). *Trauma Systems Therapy for Children and Teens*, 2nd Edn. New York: Guilford.

Ford, J., Blaustein, M., Habib, M., & Kagan, R. (2013). Developmental trauma therapy models. In J.D. Ford & C.A. Courtois (Eds) *Treating Complex Traumatic Stress Disorders in Children and Adolescents: Scientific Foundations and Therapeutic Models* (pp. 261–276). New York: Guilford Press.

Ford, J.D., & Cloitre, M. (2009). Best practices in psychotherapy for children and adolescents. In Courtois, C.A., & Ford, J.D. (Eds) *Treating Complex Traumatic Stress Disorders: An Evidence Based Guide* (pp. 59–81). New York: Guilford Press.

Ford, J.D., & Courtois, C.A. (Eds) (2013). *Treating Complex Traumatic Stress Disorders in Children and Adolescents: Scientific Foundations and Therapeutic Models*. New York: Guilford.

Ford, J.D., & Russo, E. (2006). *A trauma-focused, present-centered, emotional self-regulation approach to integrated treatment for post-traumatic stress and addiction: Trauma adaptive recovery group education and therapy (TARGET)*. American Journal of Psychotherapy, *60* (4), 335–355.

Golding, K., & McConville, J. (2014). *Using Stories to Build Bridges with Traumatized Children*. London: Jessica Kingsley Publishers.

Habib, M., Labruna, V., & Newman, J. (2013). Complex histories and complex presentations: Implementation of a manually-guided group treatment for traumatized adolescents. *Journal of Family Violence, 28*, 717–728.

Hill, R., Oosterhoff Layne, C.M., Rooney, E.E., Yudovich, S., Pynoos, R., & Kaplow, J. (2019). *Multidimensional grief therapy: Pilot open trial of a novel intervention for bereaved children and adolescents. Journal of Child and Family Studies*, https://doi.org/10.1007/s10826-019-01481-.

Howell, K.H., Shapiro, D.N., Layne, C.M., & Kaplow, J.B. (2015). Individual and psychosocial mechanisms of adaptive functioning in parentally bereaved children. *Death Studies, 39*(1–5): 296–306.

Hughes, D.A. (2007). *Attachment-Focused Family Therapy*. New York: Norton.

Hughes, D.A. (2011). *Attachment-Focused Family Therapy Workbook*. New York: Norton.

Hughes, D.A., & Baylin, J. (2012). *Brain-Based Parenting; The Neuroscience of Caregiving for Healthy Attachment*. New York: Norton.

James, B. (1994). *Handbook for Treatment of Attachment-Trauma Problems in Children*. Lexington, MA: Lexington Books.

Kagan, R. (2004). *Rebuilding Attachments with Traumatized Children: Healing from Losses, Violence, Abuse and Neglect*. New York: Routledge.

Kagan, R. (2017a). *Real Life Heroes Life Storybook*, 3rd Edn. New York: Routledge.

Kagan, R. (2017b). *Real Life Heroes Toolkit for Treating Traumatic Stress in Children and Families*, 2nd Edn. New York: Routledge.

Kagan, R. (2017c). *Wounded Angels; Inspiration from Children in Crisis*. New York: Routledge.

Kagan, R., & Spinazzola, J. (2013). *Real Life Heroes* in residential treatment: Implementation of trauma and attachment-focused treatment for children and adolescents with complex PTSD. *Journal of Family Violence, 28*(7), 705–715.

Kagan, R., Douglas, A., Hornik, J., & Kratz, S. (2008). *Real Life Heroes* pilot study: Evaluation of a treatment model for children with traumatic stress. *Journal of Child and Adolescent Trauma, 1*(1), 5–22.

Kagan, R., Henry, J., Richardson, M., Trinkle, J., & LaFrenier, A. (2014). Evaluation of *Real Life Heroes* treatment for children with complex PTSD. *Psychological Trauma: Theory, Research, Practice, and Policy, 6*(5), 588–596.

Kaplow, J.B., & Layne, C.M. (2014). Sudden loss and psychiatric disorders across the life course: Toward a developmental lifespan theory of bereavement-related risk and resilience. *American Journal of Psychiatry, 171*(8), 807–810.

Kaplow, J.B., Howell, K.H., & Layne, C.M. (2014). Do circumstances of the death matter? Identifying socioenvironmental risks for grief-related psychopathology in bereaved youth. *Journal of Traumatic Stress, 27*(1), 42–49.

Kliethermes, M., Nanney, R.W., Cohen, J.A., & Mannarino, A.P. (2013). Trauma-focused cognitive-behavioral therapy. In J.D. Ford & C.A. Courtois (Eds) *Treating Complex Traumatic Stress Disorders in Children and Adolescents: Scientific Foundations and Therapeutic Models*. New York: Guilford.

Lanktree, C.B., & Briere, J. (2016). *Treating Complex Trauma in Children and their Families: An Integrative Approach*. Thousand Oaks, CA: Sage.

Lieberman, A., & van Horn, P. (2011). *Psychotherapy with Infants and Young Children: Repairing the Effects of Stress and Trauma on Early Attachment*. New York: Guilford National Child Traumatic Stress Network, www.nctsn.org.

Perry, B.D. (2000). Traumatized children: How childhood trauma influences brain development. *The Journal of the California Alliance for the Mentally Ill, 11*(1), 48–51.

Perry, B.D. (2006). Applying principles of neurodevelopment to clinical work with maltreated and traumatized children. In N. Webb (Ed.) *Working with Traumatized Youth in Child Welfare* (pp. 27–52). New York: Guilford.

Pynoos R.S. (1992). Grief and trauma in children and adolescents. *Bereavement Care, 11*, 2–10.

Saltzman, W., Layne, C.M., Pynoos, R.S., Olafson, E., Kaplow, J.B., & Boat, B. (2013). *Trauma and Grief Component Therapy for Adolescents*. Los Angeles, University of California–Los Angeles, Department of Psychiatry and Biobehavioral Sciences.

Shapiro F. (2001). *Eye Movement Desensitization and Reprocessing: Basic Principles, Protocols, and Procedures*, 2nd Edn. New York: Guilford Press.

Siegel, D. (1999). *The Developing Mind*. New York: Guilford Press.

Siegel, D.J., & Bryson, T.P. (2011). *The Whole-Brain Child: 12 Revolutionary Strategies to Nurture Your Child's Developing Mind*. New York: Bantam Trade Paperbacks.

Solomon, M., & Siegel, D. (Eds) (2003). *Healing Trauma: Attachment, Mind, Body, and Brain*. New York: Norton.

Spinazzola, J., Habib, M., Blaustein, M., Knoverek, A., Kisiel, C., Stolbach, B., Abramovitz, R., Kagan, R., Lanktree, C., & Maze, J. (2017). *What is Complex Trauma? A Resource Guide for Youth and Those Who Care About Them.* Los Angeles, CA, and Durham, NC: National Center for Child Traumatic Stress (available at www.nctsn.org).

Straus, M. (1998). *No-Talk Therapy for Children and Adolescents*. New York: Norton.

Straus, M. (2009). Secure love: Working with adolescents and families. In M. Kerman (Ed.), *Clinical Pearls of Wisdom: Leading Therapists Offer Essential Insights*. New York: Norton.

van der Kolk, B. (2005). Developmental trauma disorder. *Psychiatric Annals*, *35*(5), 401–409.

van der Kolk, B. (2014). *The Body Keeps the Score: Brain, Mind and Body in the Healing of Trauma*. New York: Viking.

Warner, E., Cook, A., Westcott, A., & Koomar, J. (2011). *SMART: Sensory Motor Arousal Regulation Treatment.* Brookline, MA: The Trauma Center at JRI. (www.traumacenter.org/products)

Acknowledgements

The Hero's Mask novel and *Guidebook* were inspired by the children and families I've been privileged to work with over the course of my career. I have witnessed the pain of children and family members who have experienced multiple traumas. I have been inspired by the many ways that children and families have struggled to cope with these hardships. From every child and family, I have heard stories of courage and efforts to make things better. I have seen how caring and commitment by birth, foster, and adoptive parents, grandparents, teachers, residential counselors, therapists, and other caring adults can light up a child's eyes, bring out hidden talents and abilities in youths, and lead to profound changes in behavior.

I have also been privileged to learn from my colleagues in the National Child Traumatic Stress Network and at Parsons Child and Family Center and Northeast Child and Parent Society. *The Hero's Mask* includes references to research and treatment by many of my colleagues and mentors in the field of traumatic stress research including Margaret Blaustein, Sandy Bloom, John Briere, Marylene Cloitre, Julian Ford, Jim Henry, Julie Kaplow, Kristine Kinniburgh, Laurel Kiser, Cheryl Lanktree, Glenn Saxe, Patricia Van Horn, and Bessel van der Kolk, to name just a few. I am grateful to colleagues and friends who read the book and guided me to shape the story to engage children and I want to especially thank Lisa Amaya-Jackson, Margaret Blaustein, Karen Clark, Gail Darrigo, Allison Davenport-Contenelli, Karen Fein, Chandra Ghosh Ippen (and her son), Pam Howard, Robert Lominack, Sydney Madden, Margaret Richardson, and Tammi Wrest. In the final stages of writing this book, I was privileged to receive guidance and tips from Julie Kaplow, Mindy Kronenberg, Jen Maze (and her son), and my daughter, Michelle Gaines. Michelle guided reframing my book proposal and Mindy edited the novel line by line, both were a tremendous help. Cheryl Lanktree provided me with inspiration to carry on and Chandra Ghosh Ippen provided me with invaluable tips for publishing and marketing the book. I was then fortunate to be able to work with Sarah Tuckwell, editor for Routledge Education, and her staff, Will Bateman, Lucy Stewart and Jonathan Merrett. All of their help gave me the support I needed to continue writing and improving these books.

The Hero's Mask was inspired by the courage I have experienced in my family including the courage of my two fathers, my father-in-law and my uncle who fought in World War II and my grandparents and great grandparents who fled persecution in pogroms and built a better life for their children and grandchildren. My mother, Rhoda Kagan, urged me to write books from the time I was a child and taught me that there was nothing more important than raising children. I am grateful to my daughter, Michelle, for her guidance on how to promote the book and for urging me to keep working on this, to my son-in-law, Andrew Gaines for helping me to embody each character, to Gia and Amit Gupta-Kagan for giving me advice on writing the novel and guiding me to great middle grade books, and to educators in my family, Avni Gupta-Kagan, Michelle Gaines, Cindy Johnston, and Cathy Alland for their stories and guidance concerning the challenges of elementary school education. I am especially grateful to my wife, Dr. Laura Kagan, who helped me master challenges in combining a story that could engage children, provide psychoeducational content and stay true to life.

About the author

Dr. Kagan provides training and consultation on traumatic stress and complex trauma treatment and is an affiliate member of the National Child Traumatic Stress Network (NCTSN). He has had leadership experience in child and family services as the director of professional development, QI, research, and psychological services for Parsons Child and Family Center, a NCTSN community services site since 2002, and served as the principal investigator for two SAMHSA-funded NCTSN grants and as the Director of Research and Consultation for the Sidney Albert Training and Research Institute. Dr. Kagan co-led development of the NCTSN curriculum, *Caring for Children Who Have Experienced Traumatic Stress* as co-chair of the Resource Parent Committee and served on the NCTSN Steering Committee, the NCTSN Affiliate Advisory Group, the Complex Trauma and Child Welfare Committees and the advisory group for development of the NCTSN's Trauma-Informed Organizational Assessment.

Dr. Kagan's presentations, articles, and books highlight practical and innovative approaches that practitioners and organizations can utilize to help children and families strengthen resilience and reduce traumatic stress. Dr. Kagan's publications include 35+ articles and papers on practice and research issues in trauma therapy, child welfare, foster care, adoption, training implementation, program evaluation, and quality improvement and 12 books including *The Real Life Heroes Toolkit for Treating Traumatic Stress in Children and Families, The Real Life Heroes Life Storybook, Rebuilding Attachments with Traumatized Children* and *Wounded Angels; Inspiration from Children in Crisis.* Further information about Dr. Kagan's publications, training programs and professional experience can be found at www.reallifeheroes.net.

T - #0022 - 171020 - C0 - 297/210/2 - PB - 9780367474294